Table of Contents

The Vegan Diet — 3

Different Types of Vegan Diets 6

Vegan Diets Can Help You Lose Weight

.... 10

Vegan Diets, Blood Sugar and Type 2

Diabetes 13

Vegan Diets and Heart Health 15

Other Benefits of Vegan Diets 17

Foods to Avoid 20

Foods to Eat 22

Risks and How to Minimize Them ... 27

Supplements to Consider.............. 32

The Vegan Diet —

A Complete Guide for Beginners

The vegan diet has become very popular.

Increasingly more people have decided to go vegan for ethical, environmental or health reasons.

When done right, such a diet may result in various health benefits, including a trimmer waistline and improved blood sugar control.

Nevertheless, a diet based exclusively on plant foods may, in some cases, increase the risk of nutrient deficiencies.

This article is a detailed beginner's guide to the vegan diet. It aims to cover everything you need to know, so you can follow a vegan diet the right way.

What Is the Vegan Diet?

Veganism is defined as a way of living that attempts to exclude all forms of animal exploitation and cruelty, whether for food, clothing or any other purpose.

For these reasons, the vegan diet is devoid of all animal products, including meat, eggs and dairy.

People choose to follow a vegan diet for various reasons.

These usually range from ethics to environmental concerns, but they can also stem from a desire to improve health.

BOTTOM LINE:

A vegan diet excludes all animal products. Many people choose to eat this way for ethical, environmental or health reasons.

Different Types of Vegan Diets

There are different varieties of vegan diets. The most common include:

- **Whole-food vegan diet:** A diet based on a wide variety of whole plant foods such as fruits, vegetables, whole grains, legumes, nuts and seeds.

- **Raw-food vegan diet:** A vegan diet based on raw fruits, vegetables, nuts, seeds or plant foods cooked at temperatures below 118°F (48°C).

- **80/10/10:** The 80/10/10 diet is a raw-food vegan diet that limits fat-rich plants such as nuts and avocados and relies mainly on raw fruits and soft greens instead. Also referred to as the low-fat, raw-food vegan diet or fruitarian diet.

- **The starch solution:** A low-fat, high-carb vegan diet similar to the 80/10/10 but that focuses on cooked starches like potatoes, rice and corn instead of fruit.

- **Raw till 4:** A low-fat vegan diet inspired by the 80/10/10 and starch solution. Raw foods are consumed until 4 p.m., with the option of a cooked plant-based meal for dinner.

- **The thrive diet:** The thrive diet is a raw-food vegan diet. Followers eat plant-based, whole foods that are raw or minimally cooked at low temperatures.

- **Junk-food vegan diet:** A vegan diet lacking in whole plant foods that relies heavily on mock meats and cheeses, fries, vegan desserts and other heavily processed vegan foods.

Although several variations of the vegan diet exist, most scientific research rarely differentiates between different types of vegan diets.

Therefore, the information provided in this article relates to vegan diets as a whole.

BOTTOM LINE:

There are several ways to follow a vegan diet, but scientific research rarely differentiates between the different types.

Vegan Diets Can Help You Lose Weight

Vegans tend to be thinner and have a lower body mass index (BMI) than non-vegans.

This might explain why an increasing number of people turn to vegan diets as a way to lose excess weight.

Part of the weight-related benefits vegans experience may be explained by factors other than diet. These may include healthier lifestyle choices, such as physical activity, and other health-related behaviors.

However, several randomized controlled studies, which control for these external factors, report that vegan diets are more effective for weight loss than the diets they are compared to.

Interestingly, the weight loss advantage persists even when whole-food-based diets are used as control diets.

These include diets recommended by the American Dietetics Association (ADA), the American Heart Association

(AHA) and the National Cholesterol Education Program (NCEP).

What's more, researchers generally report that participants on vegan diets lose more weight than those following calorie-restricted diets, even when they're allowed to eat until they feel full.

The natural tendency to eat fewer calories on a vegan diet may be caused by a higher dietary fiber intake, which can make you feel fuller.

BOTTOM LINE:

Vegan diets seem very effective at helping people naturally reduce the amount of calories they eat, resulting in weight loss.

Vegan Diets, Blood Sugar and Type 2 Diabetes

Adopting a vegan diet may help keep your blood sugar in check and type 2 diabetes at bay.

Several studies show that vegans benefit from lower blood sugar levels, higher insulin sensitivity and up to a 78% lower risk of developing type 2 diabetes than non-vegans.

In addition, vegan diets reportedly lower blood sugar levels in diabetics up to 2.4 times more than diets recommended by the ADA, AHA and NCEP.

Part of the advantage could be explained by the higher fiber intake, which may blunt the blood sugar response. A vegan diet's weight loss effects may further contribute to its ability to lower blood sugar levels.

BOTTOM LINE:

Vegan diets seem particularly effective at improving markers of blood sugar control. They may also lower the risk of developing type 2 diabetes.

Vegan Diets and Heart Health

A vegan diet may help keep your heart healthy.

Observational studies report vegans may have up to a 75% lower risk of developing high blood pressure and 42% lower risk of dying from heart disease.

Randomized controlled studies — the gold standard in research — add to the evidence.

Several report that vegan diets are much more effective at reducing blood sugar, LDL and total cholesterol than diets they are compared to.

These effects could be especially beneficial since reducing blood pressure, cholesterol and blood sugar may reduce heart disease risk by up to 46%.

BOTTOM LINE:

Vegan diets may improve heart health. However, more high-quality studies are needed before strong conclusions can be drawn.

Other Benefits of Vegan Diets

Vegan diets are linked to an array of other health benefits, including benefits for:

- **Cancer risk:** Vegans may benefit from a 15% lower risk of developing or dying from cancer.

- **Arthritis:** Vegan diets seem particularly effective at reducing symptoms of arthritis such as pain, joint swelling and morning stiffness.

- **Kidney function:** Diabetics who substitute meat for plant protein may reduce their risk of poor kidney function.

- **Alzheimer's disease:** Observational studies show that aspects of the vegan diet may help reduce the risk of developing Alzheimer's disease.

That said, keep in mind that most of the studies supporting these benefits are observational. This makes it difficult to determine whether the vegan diet directly caused the benefits.

Randomized controlled studies are needed before strong conclusions can be made.

BOTTOM LINE:

A vegan diet is linked to several other health benefits. However, more research is needed to determine causality.

Foods to Avoid

Vegans avoid eating any animal foods, as well as any foods containing ingredients derived from animals. These include:

• Meat and poultry: Beef, lamb, pork, veal, horse, organ meat, wild meat, chicken, turkey, goose, duck, quail, etc.

• Fish and seafood: All types of fish, anchovies, shrimp, squid, scallops, calamari, mussels, crab, lobster, etc.

• Dairy: Milk, yogurt, cheese, butter, cream, ice cream, etc.

- Eggs: From chickens, quails, ostriches, fish, etc.

- Bee products: Honey, bee pollen, royal jelly, etc.

- Animal-based ingredients: Whey, casein, lactose, egg white albumen, gelatin, cochineal or carmine, isinglass, shellac, L-cysteine, animal-derived vitamin D3 and fish-derived omega-3 fatty acids.

BOTTOM LINE:

Vegans avoid consuming any animal flesh, animal byproducts or foods containing an ingredient from animal origin.

Foods to Eat

Health-conscious vegans substitute animal products with plant-based replacements, such as:

• Tofu, tempeh and seitan: These provide a versatile protein-rich alternative to meat, fish, poultry and eggs in many recipes.

• Legumes: Foods such as beans, lentils and peas are excellent sources of many nutrients and beneficial plant compounds. Sprouting, fermenting and proper cooking can increase nutrient absorption.

• Nuts and nut butters: Especially unblanched and unroasted varieties, which are good sources of iron, fiber, magnesium, zinc, selenium and vitamin E.

• Seeds: Especially hemp, chia and flaxseeds, which contain a good amount of protein and beneficial omega-3 fatty acids.

• Calcium-fortified plant milks and yogurts: These help vegans achieve their recommended dietary calcium intakes. Opt for varieties also fortified with vitamins B12 and D whenever possible.

• Algae: Spirulina and chlorella are good sources of complete protein. Other varieties are great sources of iodine.

• Nutritional yeast: This is an easy way to increase the protein content of vegan dishes and add an interesting cheesy flavor. Pick vitamin B12-fortified varieties whenever possible.

• Whole grains, cereals and pseudocereals: These are a great source of complex carbs, fiber, iron, B-vitamins and several minerals. Spelt, teff, amaranth and quinoa are especially high-protein options.

• Sprouted and fermented plant foods: Ezekiel bread, tempeh, miso, natto, sauerkraut, pickles, kimchi and kombucha often contain probiotics and vitamin K2. Sprouting and fermenting can also help improve mineral absorption.

• Fruits and vegetables: Both are great foods to increase your nutrient intake. Leafy greens such as bok choy, spinach, kale, watercress and mustard greens are particularly high in iron and calcium.

BOTTOM LINE:

These minimally processed plant foods are great additions to any vegan refrigerator or pantry.

Risks and How to Minimize Them

Favoring a well-planned diet that limits processed foods and replaces them with nutrient-rich ones instead is important for everyone, not only vegans.

That said, those following poorly planned vegan diets are particularly at risk of certain nutrient deficiencies.

In fact, studies show that vegans are at a higher risk of having inadequate blood levels of vitamin B12, vitamin D, long-chain omega-3s, iodine, iron, calcium and zinc.

Not getting enough of these nutrients is worrisome for everyone, but it may pose a particular risk to those with increased requirements, such as children or women who are pregnant or breastfeeding.

Your genetic makeup and the composition of your gut bacteria may also influence your ability to derive the nutrients you need from a vegan diet.

One way to minimize the likelihood of deficiency is to limit the amount of processed vegan foods you consume and opt for nutrient-rich plant foods instead.

Fortified foods, especially those enriched with calcium, vitamin D and vitamin B12, should also make a daily appearance on your plate.

Furthermore, vegans wanting to enhance their absorption of iron and zinc should try fermenting, sprouting and cooking foods.

Also, the use of iron cast pots and pans for cooking, avoiding tea or coffee with meals and combining iron-rich foods with a source of vitamin C can further boost iron absorption.

Moreover, the addition of seaweed or iodized salt to the diet can help vegans reach their recommended daily intake of iodine.

Lastly, omega-3 containing foods, especially those high in alpha-linolenic acid (ALA), can help the body produce longer-chain omega-3s such as eicosapentaenoic acid (EPA) and docosahexaenoic acid (DHA).

Foods high in ALA include chia, hemp, flaxseeds, walnuts and soybeans.

However, there's debate regarding whether this conversion is efficient enough to meet daily needs.

Therefore, a daily intake of 200–300 mg of EPA and DHA from an algae oil supplement may be a safer way to prevent low levels.

BOTTOM LINE:

Vegans may be at an increased risk of certain nutrient deficiencies. A well-planned vegan diet that includes nutrient-rich whole and fortified foods can help provide adequate nutrient levels.

Supplements to Consider

Some vegans may find it difficult to eat enough of the nutrient-rich or fortified foods above to meet their daily requirements.

In this case, the following supplements can be particularly beneficial:

- Vitamin B12: Vitamin B12 in cyanocobalamin form is the most studied and seems to work well for most people.

- Vitamin D: Opt for D2 or vegan D3 forms such as those manufactured by Nordic Naturals or Viridian.

- EPA and DHA: Sourced from algae oil.

- Iron: Should only be supplemented in the case of a documented deficiency. Ingesting too much iron from supplements can cause health complications and prevent the absorption of other nutrients.

- Iodine: Take a supplement or add 1/2 teaspoon of iodized salt to your diet daily.

- Calcium: Calcium is best absorbed when taken in doses of 500 mg or less at a time. Taking calcium at the same time as iron or zinc supplements may reduce their absorption.

- Zinc: Taken in zinc gluconate or zinc citrate forms. Not to be taken at the same time as calcium supplements.

BOTTOM LINE:

Vegans unable to meet their recommended nutrient intakes through foods or fortified products alone should consider taking supplements.

A Vegan Sample Menu for One Week

To help get you started, here's a simple plan covering a week's worth of vegan meals:

Monday

• Breakfast: Vegan breakfast sandwich with tofu, lettuce, tomato, turmeric and a plant-milk chai latte.

• Lunch: Spiralized zucchini and quinoa salad with peanut dressing.

• Dinner: Red lentil and spinach dal over wild rice.

Tuesday

- Breakfast: Overnight oats made with fruit, fortified plant milk, chia seeds and nuts.

- Lunch: Seitan sauerkraut sandwich.

- Dinner: Pasta with a lentil bolognese sauce and a side salad.

Wednesday

- Breakfast: Mango and spinach smoothie made with fortified plant milk and a banana-flaxseed-walnut muffin.

- Lunch: Baked tofu sandwich with a side of tomato salad.

- Dinner: Vegan chili on a bed of amaranth.

Thursday

- Breakfast: Whole-grain toast with hazelnut butter, banana and a fortified plant yogurt.

- Lunch: Tofu noodle soup with vegetables.

- Dinner: Jacket sweet potatoes with lettuce, corn, beans, cashews and guacamole.

Friday

- Breakfast: Vegan chickpea and onion omelet and a cappuccino made with fortified plant milk.

- Lunch: Vegan tacos with mango-pineapple salsa.

- Dinner: Tempeh stir-fry with bok choy and broccoli.

Saturday

- Breakfast: Spinach and scrambled tofu wrap and a glass of fortified plant milk.

- Lunch: Spiced red lentil, tomato and kale soup with whole-grain toast and hummus.

- Dinner: Veggie sushi rolls, miso soup, edamame and wakame salad.

Sunday

- Breakfast: Chickpea pancakes, guacamole and salsa and a glass of fortified orange juice.

- Lunch: Tofu vegan quiche with a side of sautéed mustard greens.

- Dinner: Vegan spring rolls.

Remember to vary your sources of protein and vegetables throughout the day, as each provides different vitamins and minerals that are important for your health.

BOTTOM LINE:

You can eat a variety of tasty plant-based meals on a vegan diet.

How to Eat Vegan at Restaurants

Dining out as a vegan can be challenging.

One way to reduce stress is to identify vegan-friendly restaurants ahead of time by using websites such as Happycow or Vegguide. Apps like VeganXpress and Vegman may also be helpful.

When dining in a non-vegan establishment, try scanning the menu online beforehand to see what vegan options they may have for you.

Sometimes, calling ahead of time allows the chef to arrange something especially for you. This permits you to arrive at the restaurant confident that you'll have something hopefully more interesting than a side salad to order.

When picking a restaurant on the fly, make sure to ask about their vegan options as soon as you step in, ideally before being seated.

When in doubt, opt for ethnic restaurants. They tend to have dishes that are naturally vegan-friendly or can be easily modified to become so.

Mexican, Thai, Middle-Eastern, Ethiopian and Indian restaurants tend to be great options.

Once in the restaurant, try identifying the vegetarian options on the menu and asking whether the dairy or eggs can be removed to make the dish vegan-friendly.

Another easy tip is to order several vegan appetizers or side dishes to make up a meal.

BOTTOM LINE: Being well prepared allows you to reduce stress when dining out as a vegan.

Healthy Vegan Snacks

Snacks are a great way to stay energized and keep hunger at bay between meals.

Some interesting, portable vegan options include:

- Fresh fruit with a dollop of nut butter

- Hummus and vegetables

- Nutritional yeast sprinkled on popcorn

- Roasted chickpeas

- Nut and fruit bars

- Trail mix

- Chia pudding

- Homemade muffins

- Whole-wheat pita with salsa and guacamole

- Cereal with plant milk

- Edamame

- Whole-grain crackers and cashew nut spread

- A plant-milk latte or cappuccino

- Dried seaweed snacks

Whenever planning a vegan snack, try to opt for fiber- and protein-rich options, which can help keep hunger away.

BOTTOM LINE:

These portable, fiber-rich, protein-rich vegan snacks are convenient options to help minimize hunger between meals.

Frequently Asked Questions

Here are some frequently asked questions about veganism.

1. Can I only eat raw food as a vegan?

Absolutely not. Although some vegans choose to do so, raw veganism isn't for everyone. Many vegans eat cooked food, and there is no scientific basis for you to eat only raw foods.

2. Will switching to a vegan diet help me lose weight?

A vegan diet that emphasizes nutritious, whole plant foods and limits processed ones may help you lose weight.

As mentioned in the weight loss section above, vegan diets tend to help people eat fewer calories without having to consciously restrict their food intake.

That said, when matched for calories, vegan diets are no more effective than other diets for weight loss.

3. What is the best milk substitute?

There are many plant-based milk alternatives to cow's milk. Soy and hemp varieties contain more protein, making them more beneficial to those trying to keep their protein intake high.

Whichever plant milk you choose, ensure it's enriched with calcium, vitamin D and, if possible, vitamin B12.

4. Vegans tend to eat a lot of soy. Is this bad for you?

Soybeans are great sources of plant-based protein. They contain an array of vitamins, minerals, antioxidants and beneficial plant compounds that are linked to various health benefits.

However, soy may suppress thyroid function in predisposed individuals and cause gas and diarrhea in others.

It's best to opt for minimally processed soy food products such as tofu and edamame and limit the use of soy-based mock meats.

Fermented soy products such as tempeh and natto are especially beneficial, as fermentation helps improve the absorption of nutrients.

5. How can I replace eggs in recipes?

Chia and flaxseeds are a great way to replace eggs in baking. To replace one egg, simply mix one tablespoon of chia or ground flaxseeds with three tablespoons of hot water and allow it to rest until it gels.

Mashed bananas can also be a great alternative to eggs in some cases.

Scrambled tofu is a good vegan alternative to scrambled eggs. Tofu can also be used in a variety of egg-based recipes ranging from omelets to frittatas and quiches.

6. How can I make sure I get enough protein?

Vegans can ensure they meet their daily protein requirements by including protein-rich plant foods in their daily meals.

7. How can I make sure I get enough calcium?

Calcium-rich foods include bok choy, kale, mustard greens, turnip greens, watercress, broccoli, chickpeas and calcium-set tofu.

Fortified plant milks and juices are also a great way for vegans to increase their calcium intake.

The RDA for calcium is 1,000 mg per day for most adults and increases to 1,200 mg per day for adults over 50 years old (73).

Some argue that vegans may have slightly lower daily requirements because of the lack of meat in their diets. Not much scientific evidence can be found to support or negate this claim.

However, current studies show that vegans consuming less than 525 mg of calcium each day have an increased risk of bone fractures.

For this reason, vegans should aim to consume 525 mg of calcium per day at the very least.

8. Should I take a vitamin B12 supplement?

Vitamin B12 is generally found in animal foods. Some plant foods may contain a form of this vitamin, but there's still debate about whether this form is active in humans.

Despite circulating rumors, there's no scientific evidence to support unwashed produce as a reliable source of vitamin B12.

The daily recommended intake is 2.4 mcg per day for adults, 2.6 mcg per day during pregnancy and 2.8 mcg per day while breastfeeding.

Vitamin B12-fortified products and supplements are the only two reliable forms of vitamin B12 for vegans.

Unfortunately, many vegans seem to fail to consume sufficient vitamin B12 to meet their daily requirements.

If you're unable to meet your daily requirements through the use of vitamin B12-fortified products, you should definitely consider taking a vitamin B12 supplement.

Take Home Message

Individuals may choose veganism for ethical, environmental or health reasons.

When done right, the vegan diet can be easy to follow and may provide various health benefits.

As with any diet, these benefits only appear if you are consistent and build your diet around nutrient-rich plant foods rather than heavily processed ones.

Vegans, especially those who are unable to meet their daily nutrient requirements through diet alone, should consider supplements.